Understa

AIDS

A SELF-DEFENCE MANUAL

Whilst the author has made every effort to present objective and up-to-date information, the subject matter of this book is such that neither he nor the publisher can accept responsibility for the accuracy of its contents.

Understanding AIDS

A Self-Defence Manual

CHRISTOPHER ROUAN

Ryburn Publishing

Ryburn Publishing
Krumlin, Halifax, England

First Published 1987

Typeset by Manor Typesetting, Bradford.
Designed by Long & Stebbens Graphic Design, Bradford.
Printed and bound by The Blackmore Press, Shaftesbury, Dorset.

ISBN 1-85331-001-8

Christopher Rouan has been professionally involved in education since graduating in zoology in 1973. His major interest today is the human and social biology of health-related issues which, with his clear, sensitive and direct style of presentation, makes him an ideal guide to the complex subject matter of this widely-researched book. He is co-author of Basic Biology Questions for GCSE.

Introduction

AIDS – Acquired Immune Deficiency Syndrome – is a condition caused by the Human Immunodeficiency Virus (HIV or AIDS virus for short). The AIDS virus reduces the body's ability to resist invasion by the wide range of microscopic organisms, such as bacteria, fungi and viruses, which cause disease. These microbes affect in particular the digestive system, lungs, nervous system and skin. Cancers may also develop. The condition is incurable and fatal, and a safe preventative vaccine ready for general use is unlikely to be produced before the year 2000.

AIDS has come to be recognised as one of the greatest threats to public health this century. Consequently there has been a rapid and radical reappraisal of education in this sensitive and controversial area. Some people may be shocked or offended by the open and frank nature of the discussions, which necessarily entail public consideration of the details of sexual practices. But most research suggests that an increase in public knowledge and awareness is already beginning to have a beneficial effect. For example, the incidence of sexually transmitted diseases has reduced among the homosexual communities. As with many other diseases, a clear understanding of AIDS is one of the best means of self-defence.

Contents

1. Viruses
2. Immunity
3. The History of AIDS
4. The Signs and Symptoms of AIDS
5. The Spread of the Disease
6. Avoiding AIDS: Control and Prevention
7. The Care of AIDS Patients
8. The Development of a Vaccine

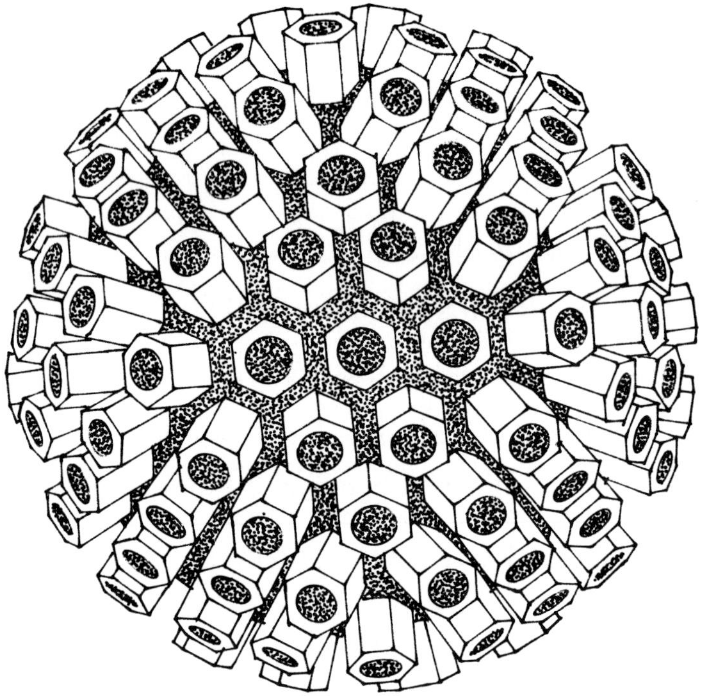

HERPES VIRUS

1. Viruses

Viruses are the smallest living organisms known to man. They were discovered to cause disease just under a hundred years ago but scientists were not able to observe their structure until much more recently. They are too small to be seen with an ordinary microscope so it was not until the development of the far more powerful electron microscope in the early 1940's that their details were revealed.

Their size is measured in units called nanometres; a nanometre is one millionth of a millimetre. A typical virus measures about 100 nanometres, which is about 50 times smaller than a bacterium. Approximately 10,000,000,000 can fit on a single pin head.

They appear in a variety of shapes: some are simple coiled rods; others such as the AIDS virus are many-sided but generally spherical; and a few, like the pox virus, are much more complex.

In structure viruses are simpler than any other living organism. They consist of a coiled length of nucleic acid, either DNA (deoxyribonucleic acid) or RNA (ribonucleic acid). This forms the core which is surrounded by a symmetrical shell of protein called a capsid. In common with herpes viruses, the AIDS virus is surrounded by an extra coat or envelope. This is formed from the membrane of the living body cell in which the virus is actively growing.

THESE DIAGRAMS SHOW THE WIDE RANGE OF VIRUS FORMS

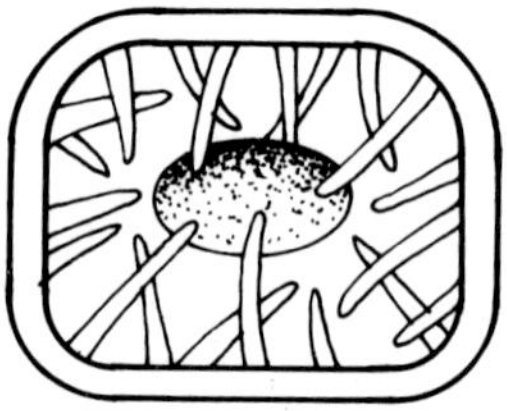

VACCINIA VIRUS

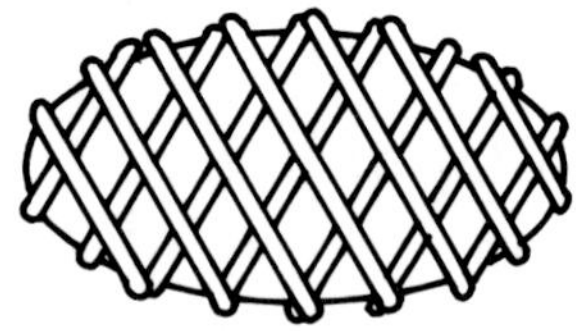

POX VIRUS

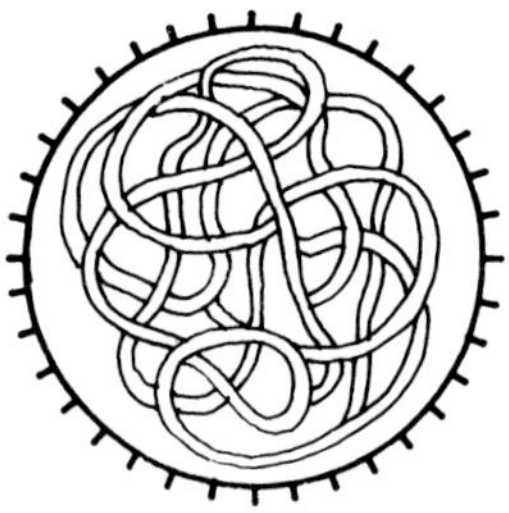

MUMPS VIRUS

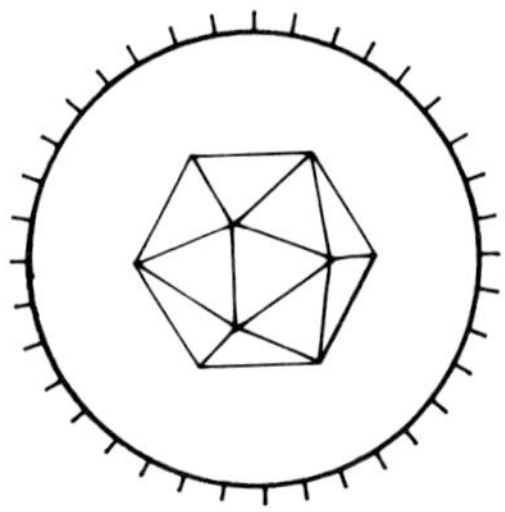

HERPES VIRUS

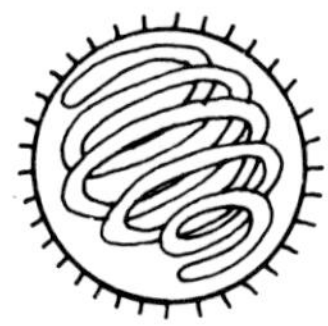

INFLUENZA VIRUS

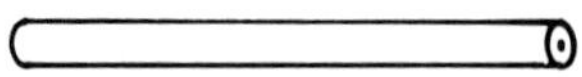

TOBACCO MOSAIC VIRUS

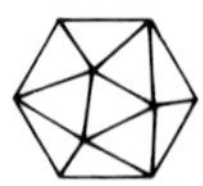

ADENO VIRUS

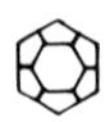

POLIO VIRUS

Viruses are completely parasitic and can reproduce only inside the cells of other living organisms.

Their life-cycle is quite remarkable and it helps to explain why they can be so devastating in their effect.

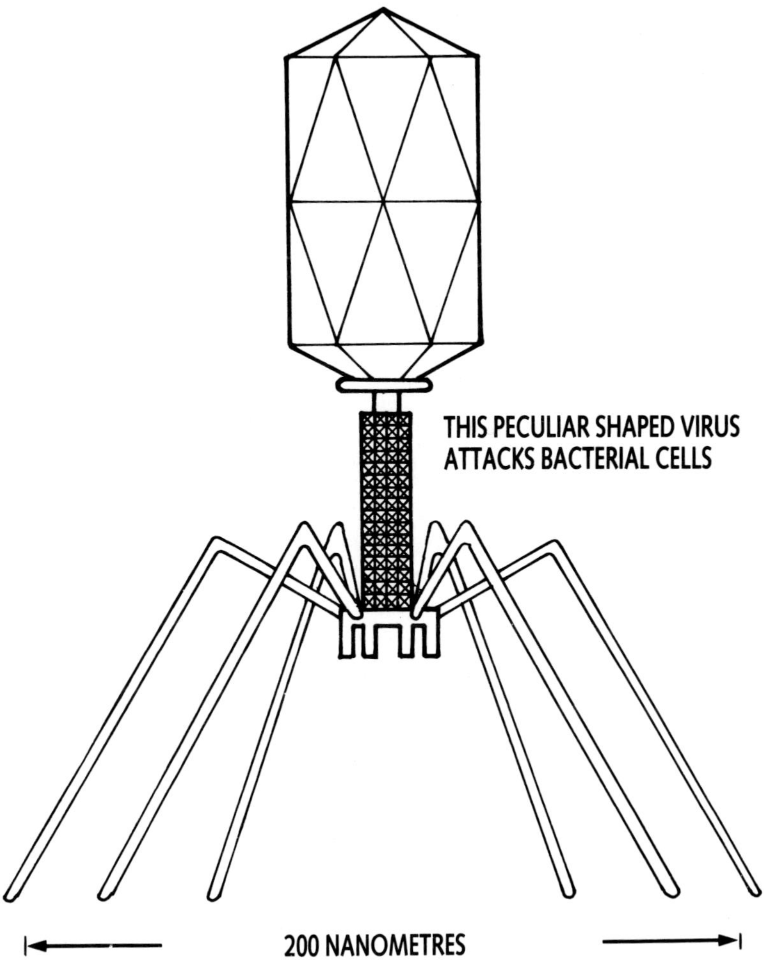

THE GENERALISED FEATURES OF A VIRUS

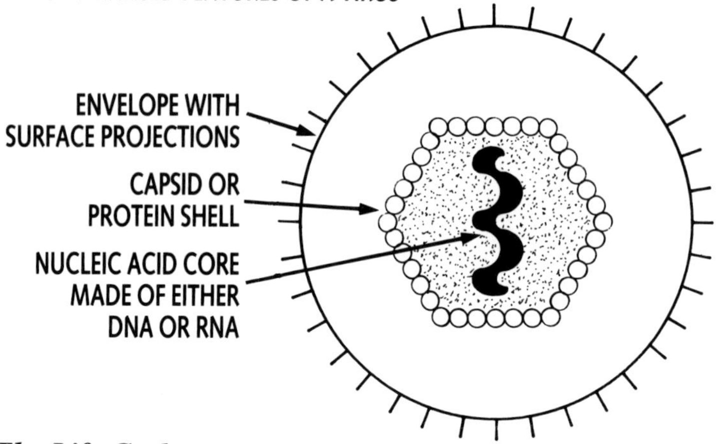

The Life-Cycle

1. The virus attaches itself to the surface of a body cell.
2. The virus enters the cell.
3. The virus takes over and destroys the cell, using it to produce and assemble thousands of new viruses.
4. The mature viruses are released, ready to infect and destroy other body cells.

Some viruses reproduce rapidly but others remain dormant in cells for years, reproducing only when faced with abnormal or suddenly changing conditions. Different viruses attack different cells. The common cold virus, for example, invades only the cells lining the nose and throat. The AIDS virus invades certain white blood cells and some nerve tissue. The fact that viruses are parasitic and live inside the cells of a host makes them very difficult to attack. The body does not normally react against and destroy its own cells.

THE VIRUS LIFE CYCLE

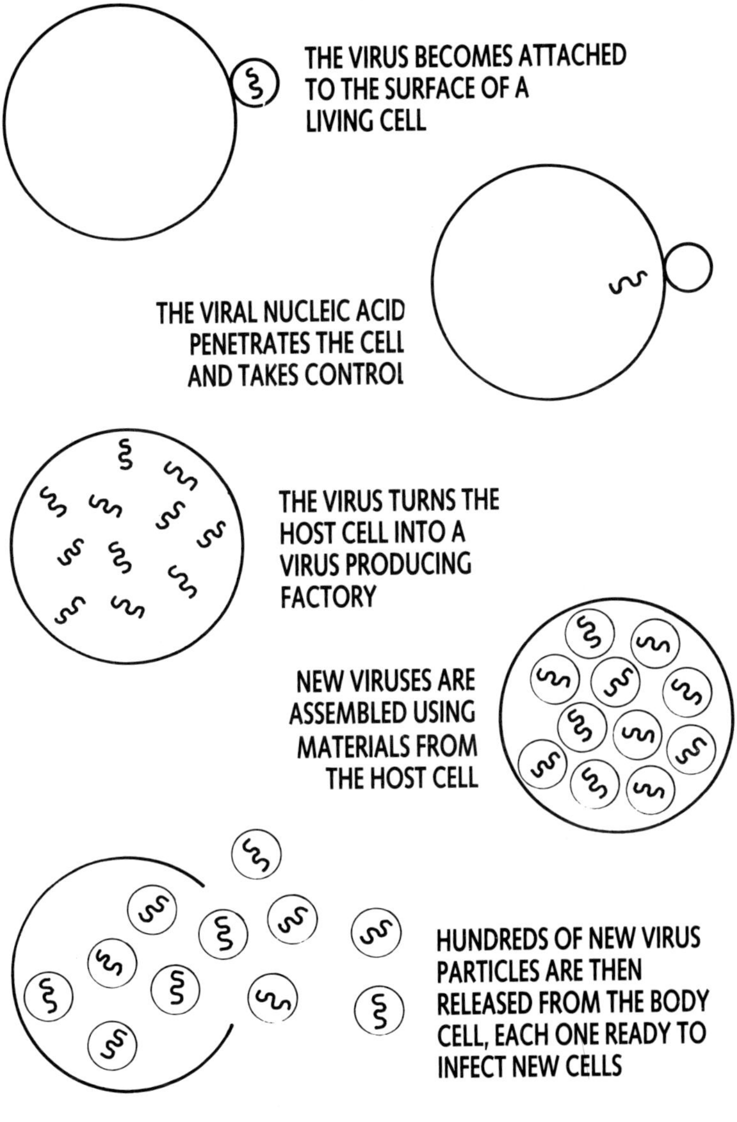

2. *Immunity*

Since the AIDS virus kills its victims by destroying their immune system, it is important to appreciate how a normal immune response helps us to survive constant invasion by microbes.

In summary, immunity refers to the body's ability to distinguish between its own protein and the foreign or antigenic protein of an invading organism. Once recognised the antigen is rejected and destroyed. This usually involves the release of specific antibodies, which are produced by special types of white blood cell called lymphocytes.

We all play host to large numbers of bacteria, viruses and protozoa, chiefly on the skin and in the gut. But it is by no means easy for harmful micro-organisms to invade or survive inside the human body.

First, there is the problem of entry. The skin which covers the body is a thick tough barrier producing an antiseptic oil, sebum. The nose filters out dirty particles from the air and the acid secreted by the stomach effectively kills many bacteria. The reproductive and respiratory tracts are lined with tiny hairs which beat and create currents, driving out invading micro-organisms. If blood vessels are broken through injury, a blood clot forms and seals off the tissues.

THE FIRST LINE OF DEFENCE AGAINST INVADING MICROBES

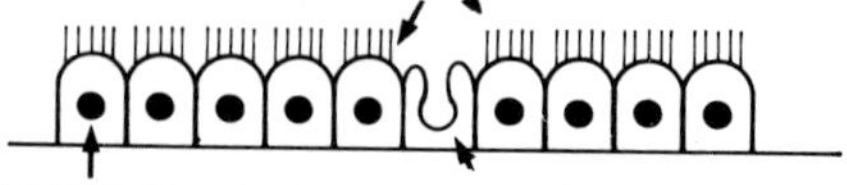
CILIA BEAT TO AND FRO
CREATING A CURRENT
THESE CELLS LINE THE
RESPIRATORY TRACT
MUCUS
PRODUCING CELL

THE WINDPIPE AND TUBES LEADING TO THE LUNGS ARE PROTECTED BY CILIA AND MUCUS WHICH TRAP GERMS

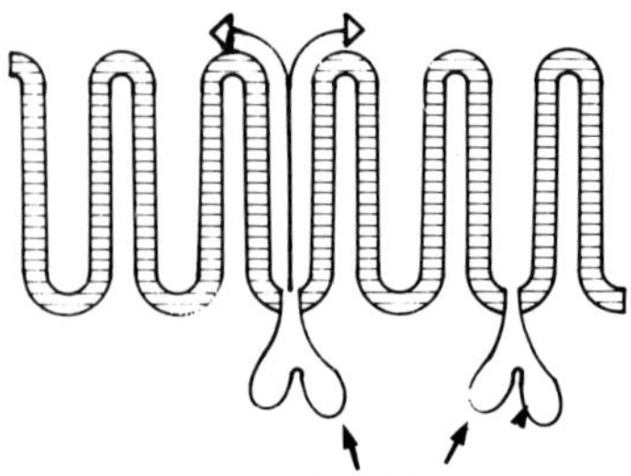

THE STOMACH WALL CONTAINS GLANDS WHICH PRODUCE ACID AND DIGESTIVE JUICES

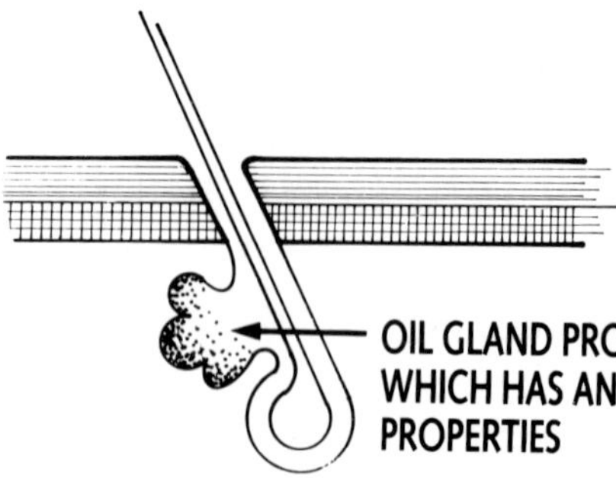

THE SKIN IS VERY THICK AND HAS MANY LAYERS OF CELLS. IT IS WATERPROOF AND SELF-REPAIRING

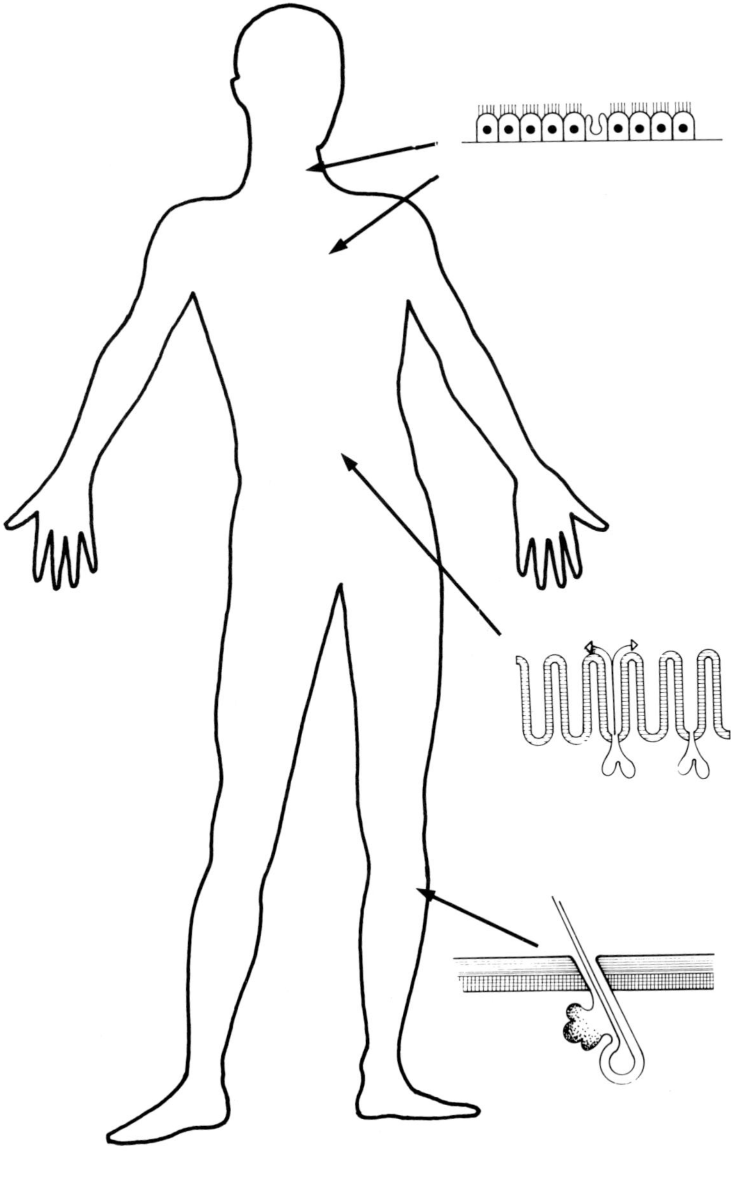

If the body's first lines of defence are penetrated, then a formidable attack on the invaders takes place: this is the immune response.

The body's internal defence against disease is mainly blood based, and although in appearance blood looks like a simple liquid, it is in fact a very special type of tissue. It consists of many cells floating about in a fluid called the plasma.

Broadly, there are two types of cells:

1) *Red blood cells* contain the red pigment haemoglobin and are responsible for carrying oxygen around the body.

2) *White blood cells* are concerned with killing germs and producing antibodies, thus helping to defend the body against disease. These are some of the cells attacked and destroyed by the AIDS virus.

All blood cells are made in the bone marrow and there are approximately 700 red cells for every white cell.

The white cells can be divided into two main types:

1) *Phagocytes* – these feed directly on invading germs by engulfing and digesting them. Phagocytes are constantly patrolling the body on the look out for invading microbes.

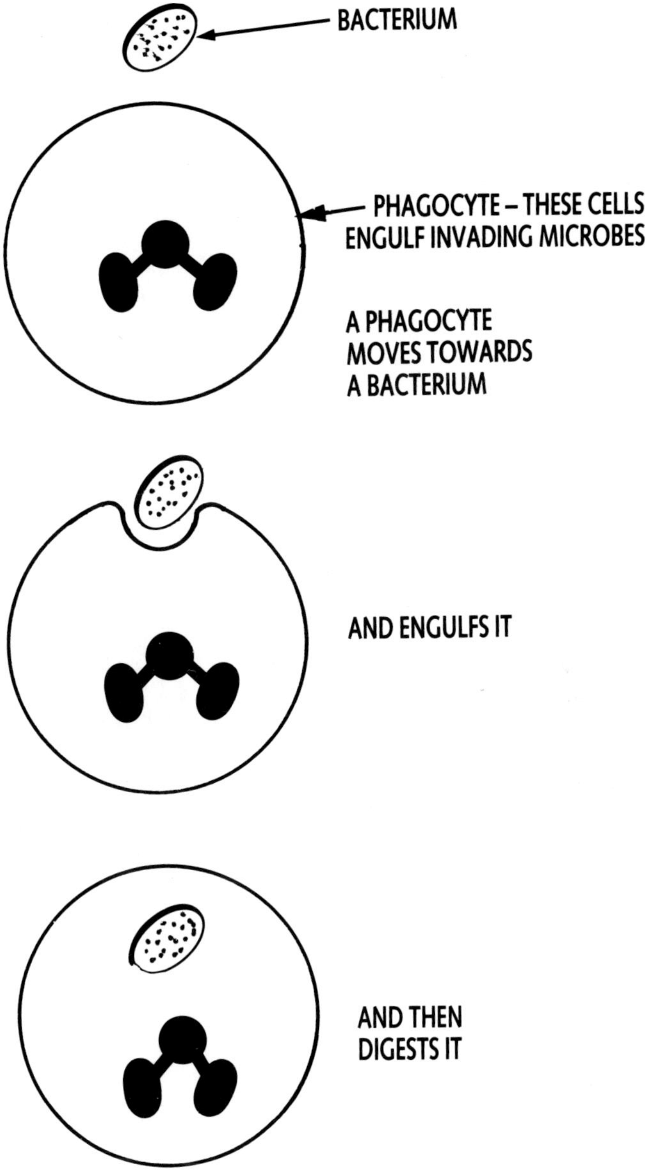
BACTERIUM
PHAGOCYTE – THESE CELLS ENGULF INVADING MICROBES
A PHAGOCYTE MOVES TOWARDS A BACTERIUM
AND ENGULFS IT
AND THEN DIGESTS IT

2) *Lymphocytes* – these cells respond in a more complex way to the germs which enter our body. They are able to recognise the virus or bacterium as an invader. This is usually because the outer coating of the germs contain chemicals which are recognised as foreign and not a normal part of the body. These chemicals are antigens: when antigens get into the body, some lymphocytes respond by attaching themselves to the antigen. They then send messages to other lymphocytes signalling them to produce special proteins called antibodies. The antibodies combine with the antigens, killing the germ.

SMALL LYMPHOCYTE

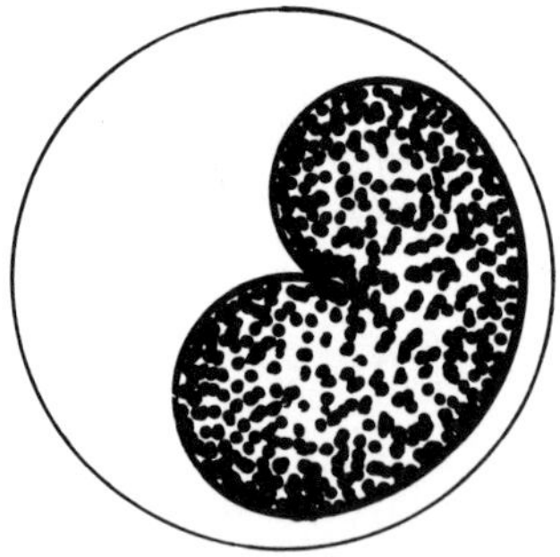

LARGE LYMPHOCYTE

THESE CELLS HELP TO PRODUCE ANTIBODIES

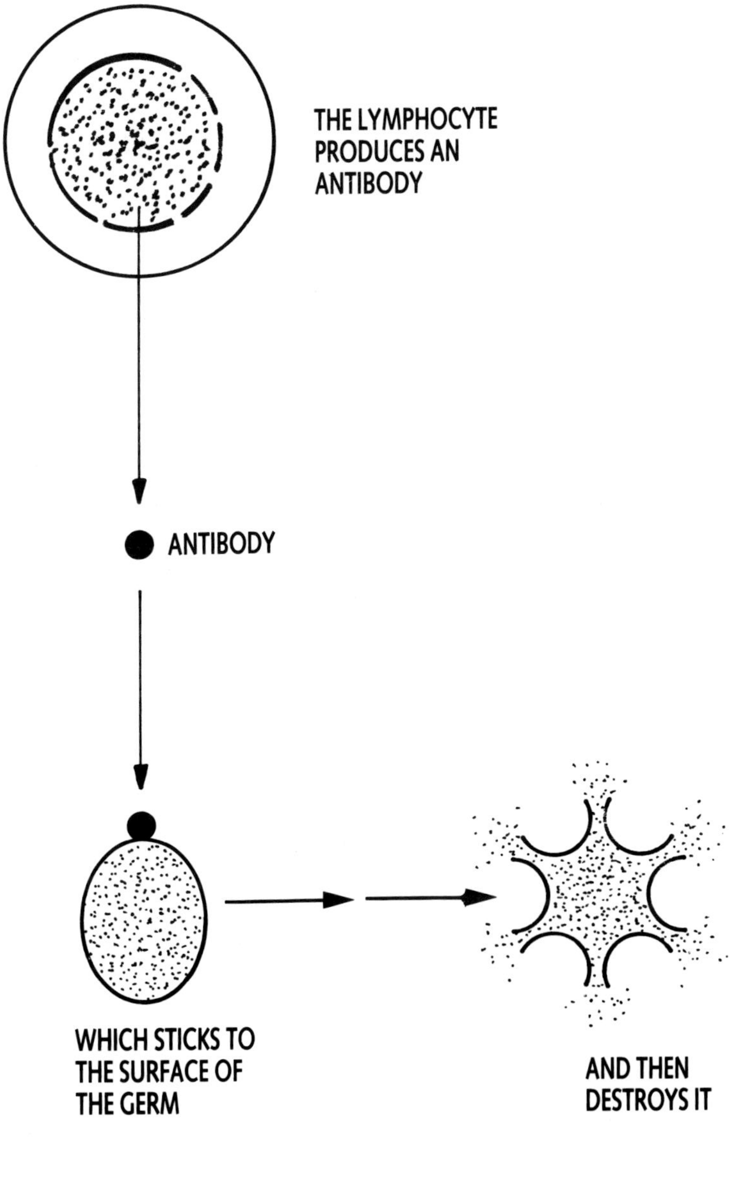
THE LYMPHOCYTE
PRODUCES AN
ANTIBODY
ANTIBODY
WHICH STICKS TO
THE SURFACE OF
THE GERM
AND THEN
DESTROYS IT

Any substance, from whatever source, which stimulates the production of antibodies is called an antigen. Viruses (including the AIDS virus), bacteria and most of their poisonous products are antigens.

Antibodies are also known to be specific, which means that each type of antibody can only combine with one type of antigen and no other. For example, the antibody against the polio virus antigen will destroy this specific virus but will have no effect on any other type of virus or bacterium.

Clearly the body must be able to produce many different antibodies in order to combat each type of antigen. This is the role of the lymphocytes. Large numbers of lymphocytes are found in special glands called lymph nodes. These glands can become inflamed when we are ill.

The way the microbes are killed varies from one kind of antibody to another. Some antibodies stick to the surface of microbes, making it easier for the phagocytes to engulf them; others stick the microbes together; and some cause the microbes to burst. If the microbes release poisons, then antibodies can combine with the chemicals to make them harmless. These antibodies are called antitoxins.

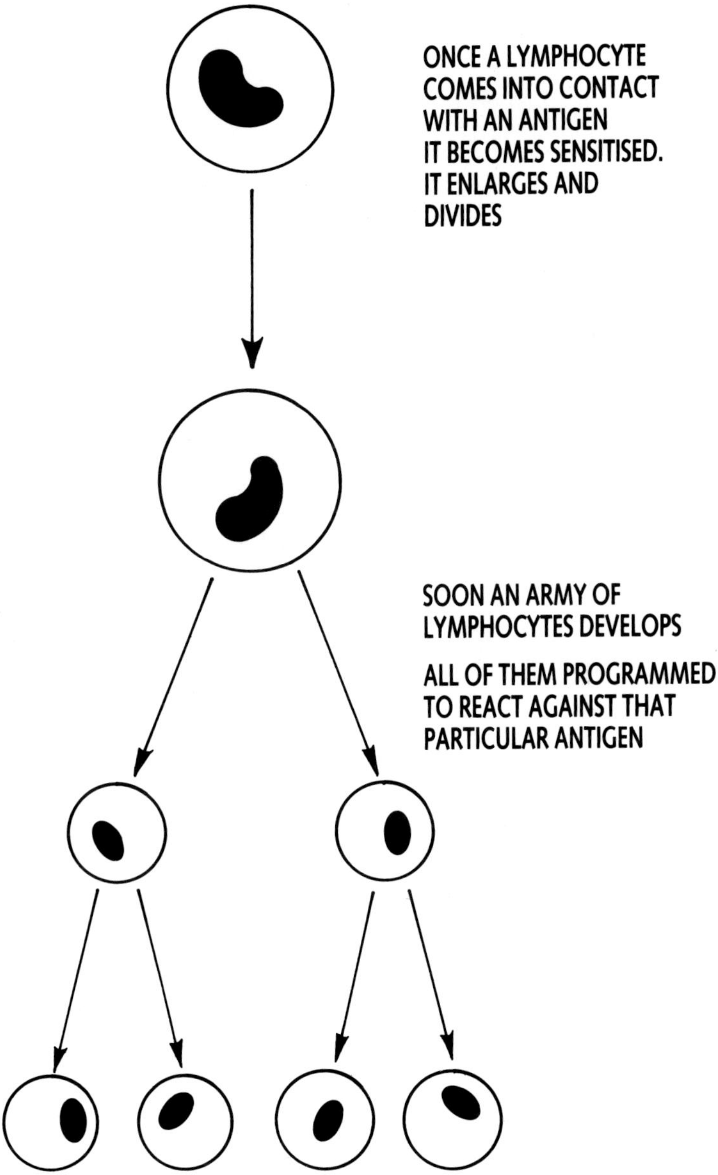
ONCE A LYMPHOCYTE
COMES INTO CONTACT
WITH AN ANTIGEN
IT BECOMES SENSITISED.
IT ENLARGES AND
DIVIDES
SOON AN ARMY OF
LYMPHOCYTES DEVELOPS
ALL OF THEM PROGRAMMED
TO REACT AGAINST THAT
PARTICULAR ANTIGEN

3. The History of AIDS

The first clinically recognised cases of AIDS were reported in the United States in 1981. A number of previously healthy homosexual men developed a serious lung infection, Pneumocystis carinii, a rare form of pneumonia. In the same year a group of similarly healthy homosexual men were found to be suffering from a rare form of skin cancer, Kaposi's sarcoma.

Both these illnesses were known to develop only in patients whose immune systems were defective. Somehow the capability of these men to produce antibodies to attack and kill invading germs had been severely and permanently damaged. The condition was called Acquired Immune Deficiency Syndrome, and as the name suggests, it can be passed from one person to another, and it kills its victims by destroying the immune system. It is now known to be caused by a virus, which was identified in 1983 by Montagnier and colleagues at the Pasteur Institute in Paris.

The virus has been called various names – Human T-cell Lymphotropic Virus type III by the Americans, Lymphadenopathy Associated Virus by the French. The International Committee on the Taxonomy of Viruses recently agreed to rename the virus Human Immunodeficiency Virus – HIV.

Since the disease was first recognised, the number of

cases has risen alarmingly, doubling every six to twelve months in Europe and the USA. In the UK there are thought to be over 40,000 people who have so far become infected with the virus, 700 have developed the symptoms, and over 300 of these have died (March 1987). Of all the 100 or so countries affected by AIDS, America has by far the worst problem; over 26000 people have developed the symptoms and over 15000 have died (December 1986). These are truly frightening statistics.

Recently it has been confirmed that AIDS-type illnesses discovered in Africa are caused by the same virus as those in Europe and the USA. Indeed in some African cities up to a quarter of the population are infected with the AIDS virus. However it is difficult to gain an accurate overall picture on the spread of AIDS in Africa since there are few researchers working on the problem, and the keeping of clinical records has been a low priority. AIDS has also been reported in Central and South America, Canada and Australasia.

The notion that the AIDS virus was manufactured in a germ-warfare laboratory has been largely discredited. Frozen blood samples from a person living in Zaire in 1959 have been found to contain traces of antibodies to the AIDS virus. This is strong evidence that the virus existed in 1959 and long before scientists had perfected the genetic engineering techniques they would have needed to create such a virus. However the

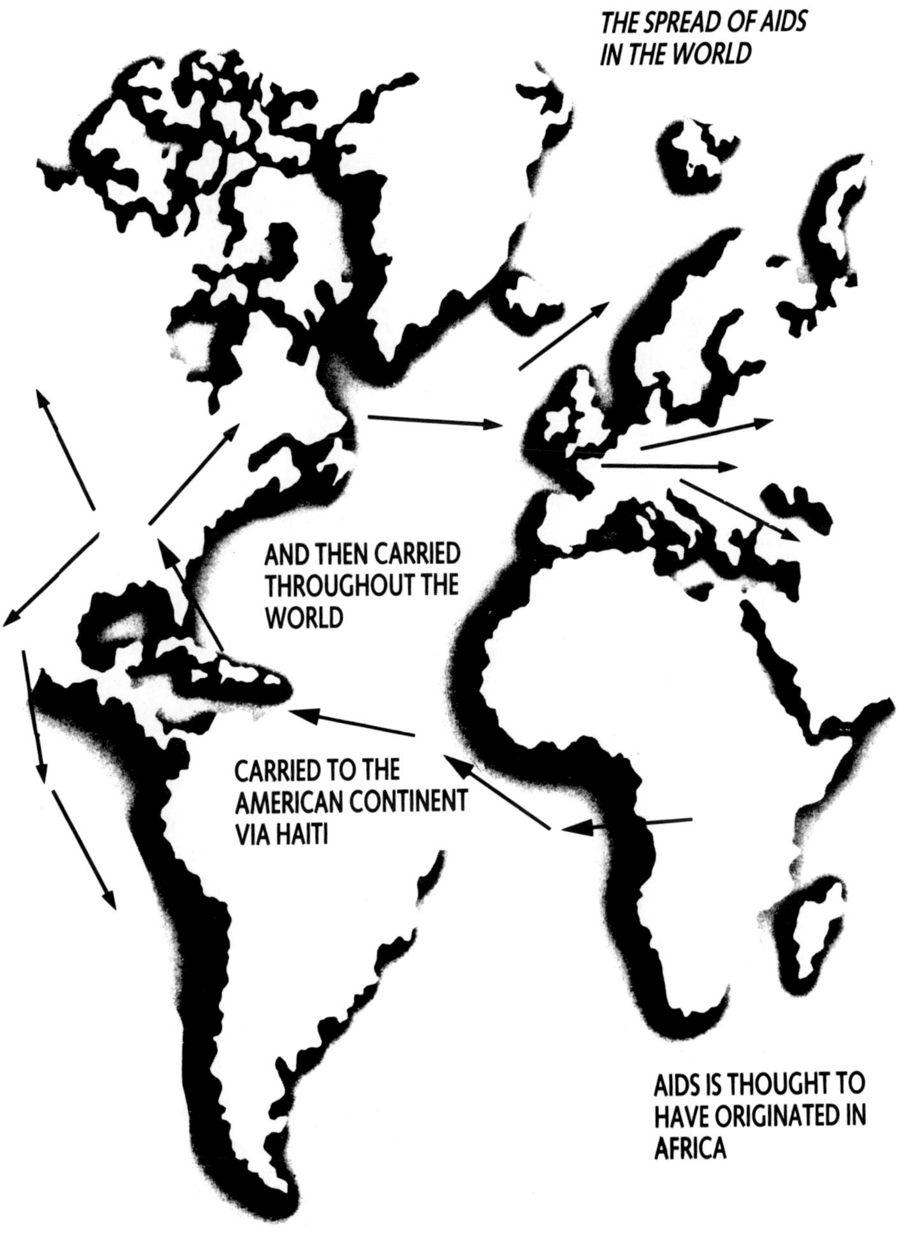
THE SPREAD OF AIDS
IN THE WORLD
AND THEN CARRIED
THROUGHOUT THE
WORLD
CARRIED TO THE
AMERICAN CONTINENT
VIA HAITI
AIDS IS THOUGHT TO
HAVE ORIGINATED IN
AFRICA

whole question of whether AIDS originated in Africa continues to be a matter of uncertainty and controversy.

There are many different types of viruses and the Human Immunodeficiency Virus has been classified as a retrovirus. These are mainly animal viruses and have been discovered in humans only during the last six years. The virus has been found in monkeys and it is thought that the disease may have been transmitted to humans through a bite. There have been recent reports from America claiming discovery of a 'sister' AIDS virus in cats.

The AIDS virus has three important characteristics:

1) Unlike other retroviruses it has a high reproductive rate which means that cells in the body are affected very quickly.

2) The AIDS virus changes its genetic structure over time, even within an individual. Its rate of evolution is much greater than for most organisms.

3) The protein structure of its outer coating or envelope is variable. This makes specific antibody production a serious problem.

Retroviruses are attracted to special white blood cells, called T-lymphocytes, which play a central role in the production of antibodies. The body's defences are thus the first victim of the AIDS virus as it invades and lives inside the very cells which are out to destroy it. Without these cells, the body is susceptible to a whole range of infections to which it is normally resistant.

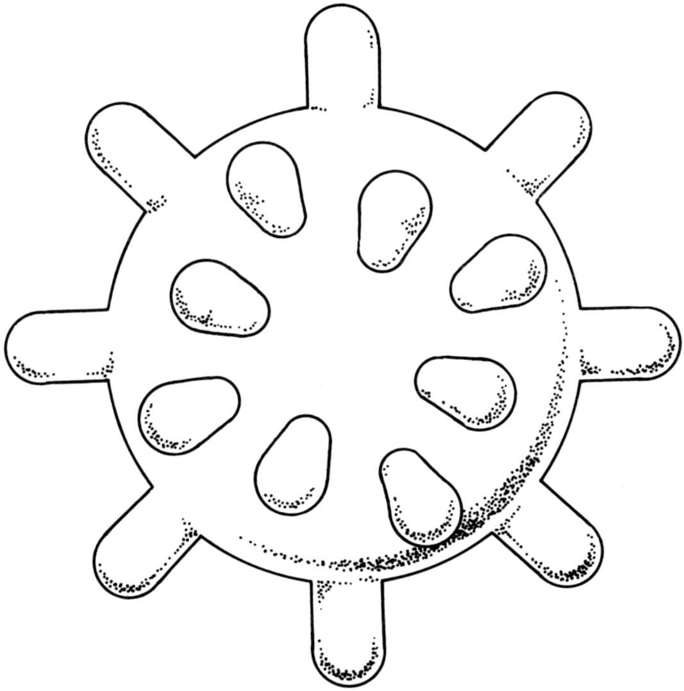

The AIDS virus

4. The Signs and Symptoms of AIDS

In its early stages AIDS is a difficult disease to diagnose directly since the symptoms are variable and not unusual.

There can be many reasons why such symptoms appear which have nothing to do with AIDS. For example, feverishness and fatigue frequently herald a bout of 'flu. Swollen lymph glands may be a sign of mumps or glandular fever. For most people AIDS will be among the least likely causes of any such symptoms. Only if the symptoms occur together and last for much longer than usual may AIDS be suspected as a possible cause.

The AIDS virus attacks the body's immune system which normally protects us from invading microbes. Our immune system responds to this virus by producing anti-AIDS virus antibody. This unfortunately has little effect on the virus which continues to attack the immune system.

Depending on the damage to the body's immune system, some people may remain quite healthy. Others may suffer one or more illnesses, usually caused directly by the virus. This is known as the AIDS Related Complex and here none of the more serious opportunistic infections or cancers are found. These patients usually suffer from swollen lymph glands, night sweats, fever and weight loss.

As the immune system is destroyed, the body is further weakened by a series of opportunistic infections. These are crippling and fatal infections to which the body is normally completely resistant. Many of them are caused by organisms, some recently discovered in humans, which usually live quite harmlessly inside the body. This is AIDS.

Five major organ systems can be affected by the AIDS syndrome:

1. The Lungs – Over 60% of AIDS patients suffer from pneumonia. It is usually caused by a protozoan parasite, Pneumocystis carinii, and is the most common cause of death.

2. The Gastrointestinal Tract – Chronic diarrhoea is a frequent symptom of the AIDS syndrome. A severe internal form of the fungal infection 'thrush' can develop. Ulcers caused by the Herpes simplex (cold sore) virus also appear internally and may spread to the skin and genitals. This can be very painful.

3. The Nervous System – Fungal infections and cancers may develop in the brain and spinal cord. Dementia, depression, seizures and a rare form of meningitis are frequently seen in AIDS patients. Viral infections can result in memory loss and eventual coma. Symptoms affecting the nervous system can be particularly distressing.

THESE ARE REGIONS WHICH IN ADDITION TO THE SKIN ARE PARTICULARLY AFFECTED DURING THE DEVELOPMENT OF AIDS

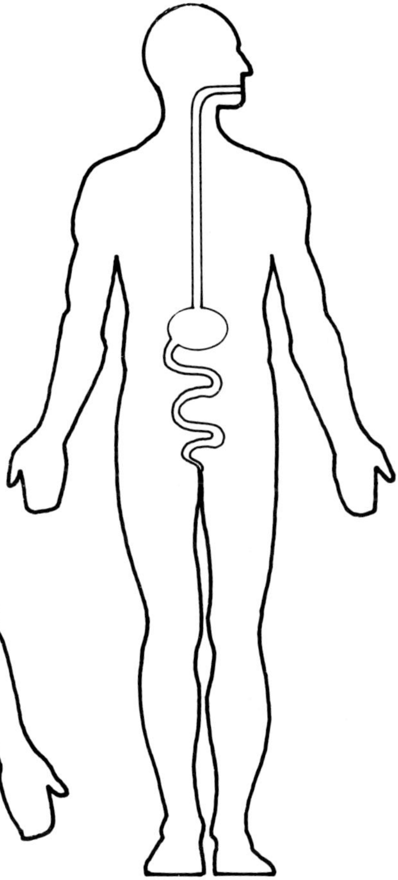

GASTRO-INTESTINAL TRACT

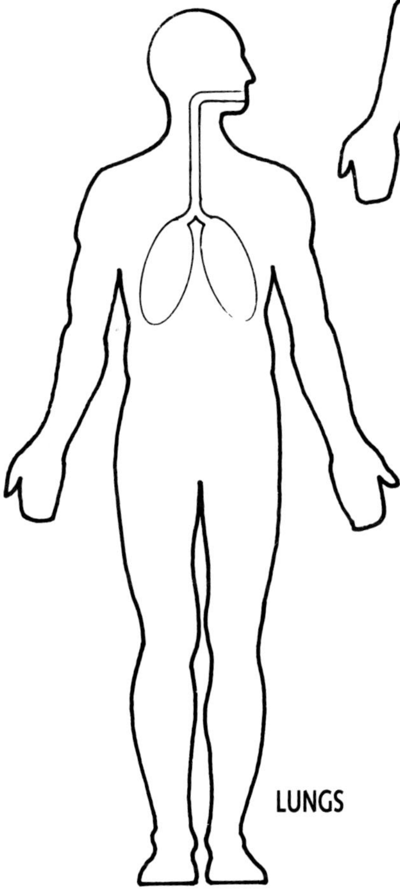

LUNGS

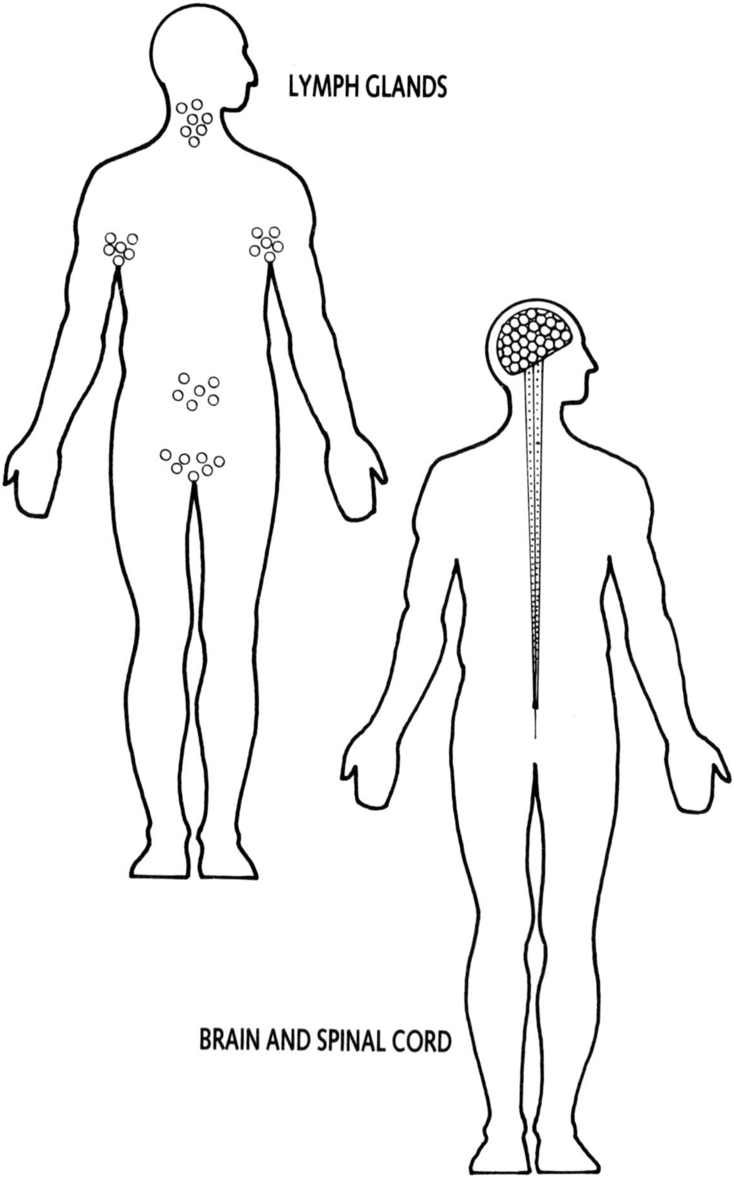
LYMPH GLANDS
BRAIN AND SPINAL CORD

4. *The Skin* – The normally rare form of skin cancer, Kaposi's sarcoma, is commonly identified in AIDS patients – more than one in four patients with AIDS develop this cancer. In the early stages it looks like the pink/purple blotches of bruising. But unlike bruises the blotches may remain, become larger, and spread. They may occur anywhere on the body including the mouth and eyelids.

5. *The Lymph Nodes* – These are persistently inflamed and occasionally infected with fungi.

In 1986 the World Health Organisation defined two levels of diagnosis depending on the facilities available.

The formal definition of a case of AIDS must show the following features:

i) the patient must be suffering from at least one of the opportunistic diseases previously described;

ii) there is no cause for the damaged immune system other than infection by the AIDS virus.

This would be supported by laboratory tests confirming the presence of the virus and/or the antibody. Blood cell counts would reveal changes in the populations of the T-lymphocytes. All this would lead to a conclusive diagnosis.

In countries where facilities are limited, a provisional clinical diagnosis would be based upon:

i) at least two of the following major symptoms –

diarrhoea (usually chronic and lasting for more than a month)
fever and night sweating (lasting for more than a month)
unexpected loss of weight (at least 10% of the body weight);

ii) at least one of the following minor symptoms –

persistent dry cough (lasting for more than a month)
swollen lymph nodes (especially in the neck and armpits)
thrush (infecting the mouth and throat)
shingles (recurrent Herpes zoster)
cold sores (chronic and progressive infection of Herpes simplex).

The presence of Kaposi's sarcoma alone is often sufficient for a positive diagnosis of AIDS.

The death rate in confirmed AIDS patients is very high. Over 50% die within a year of diagnosis, a further 30% die within the next two to three years.

However, the time between infection and the development of symptoms is very variable, from eight months to at least six years. The pattern of the disease has been followed for only the past six years therefore no-one can yet say how many of those infected will go on to realise the symptoms. So far in the UK about

30% of those known to be carrying the virus have developed the AIDS Related Complex and a further 10% have developed AIDS. There are professional predictions that possibly all those infected with the AIDS virus will eventually develop the syndrome.

As with many diseases, some people are more susceptible to illness than others. For a few this may be due to an inherited strength or weakness, but for most people the reason remains unclear. This is also true in the case of AIDS: no-one really knows why some people develop symptoms of the disease earlier than others.

However it is well known that a healthy life-style can help the body to resist disease. A sensible balance of exercise and relaxation, a nourishing diet, no smoking, and a restricted intake of alcohol are important considerations. Needless to say drug-abuse with its associated problems can often weaken considerably the body's defences against disease.

5. *The Spread of the Disease*

It is probably the spread of the AIDS virus which has attracted more media coverage than any other aspect of the disease. Whilst some has been factually correct, much has been irresponsibly exaggerated, with the result that myths and unfounded fears have mushroomed.

Although AIDS is infectious it is not very contagious, and compared to say chicken pox or the common cold, it is a very difficult disease to catch. The AIDS virus is rather fragile and can survive only in body fluids, whereas the cold virus, for example, is much more resistant and can survive outside the body for some time. This helps to explain why colds are so easily spread from one person to another as the infective virus particles are carried in the air.

The AIDS virus has been found in bone marrow cells, whole blood, plasma, lymph glands, spinal fluid, brain tissue, saliva, semen, tears and vaginal secretions.

As far as we know, it is possible for an uninfected person to catch AIDS only by the intimate exchange of body fluids with a person carrying the AIDS virus. Such a means of transmission is by no means unique to AIDS. There are many other diseases, such as rabies, syphilis and infectious hepatitis, which depend upon the intimate contact and exchange of body fluids to pass effectively from one host to another. In the case of AIDS it is only blood and semen which have been shown to be infective. Blood to blood and semen to blood contacts should therefore be avoided.

There has been one case reported recently where a patient contracted AIDS through donor skin-graft tissue. The authorities are now fully alerted to this risk, which in any event is minimal as most skin used in grafting comes directly from the patient's own body.

No-one so far as we know has caught AIDS through saliva or tears. Clearly if saliva were involved there would be far more cases of AIDS than there are at the moment, the pattern of the epidemic would be completely different, and the doctors and nurses treating and caring for AIDS patients would be at a very much greater risk than they have been shown to be.

Sexual intercourse

By its very nature sexual intercourse involves the exchange of body fluids – the passing of semen from one partner to the other. However, as internal fertilisation has evolved through the various animal groups, so has a rather elaborate and largely effective defence system. In humans the vagina is protected from invading germs in several ways. It has a thick lining composed of many layers of cells which helps to prevent microbes penetrating the body. The walls of

THE MALE REPRODUCTIVE ORGANS
SIDE VIEW

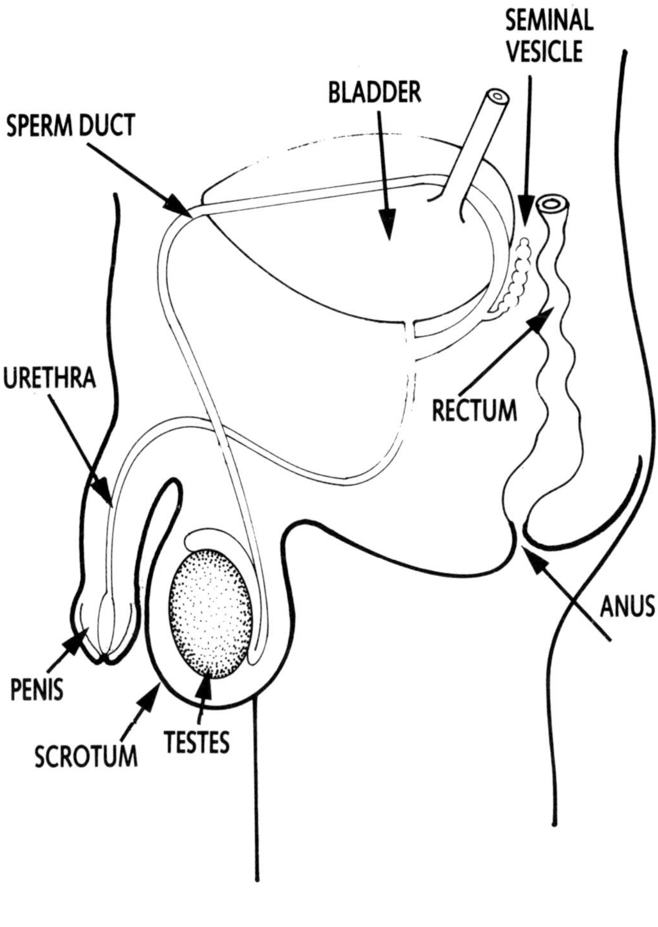

THE FEMALE REPRODUCTIVE ORGANS SIDE VIEW

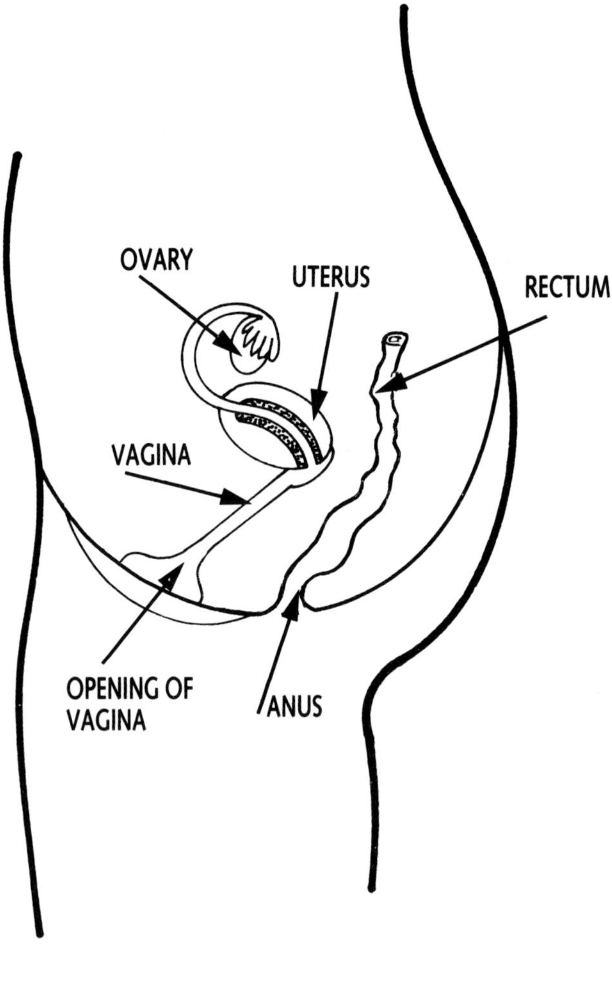

the vagina are muscular and folded: the ability to stretch without tearing or bleeding is an essential design feature since the vagina has to receive the penis during intercourse and also form part of the birth canal. The mucus secretions of the vagina are acidic and this prevents the growth of bacteria.

Therefore during vaginal intercourse there would not normally be any direct contact between semen and blood. However, the fact that the AIDS virus can be transmitted in this way suggests that somehow it is able to break through the initial vaginal defences.

Here of course it is not alone and diseases such as gonorrhoea, syphilis, genital herpes and non-specific urethritis are well-established and familiar. It has been suggested that the presence of one or more of these venereal diseases may assist the invasion of the AIDS virus.

The isolation of the AIDS virus from vaginal secretions suggests that it may pass not only from male to female but also from female to male.

During sexual arousal the blood vessels in the penis and vagina dilate and move closer to the surface. It is thought that this makes it easier for the AIDS virus to pass from one partner to another, either through the vaginal lining, through the skin of the penis, or through the urethra, the tube along which urine passes. Any inflammation caused by other infections will also ease the passage of the virus.

RECTUM

This delicate layer of cells is designed to absorb water and secrete mucus. They are easily damaged during anal intercourse.

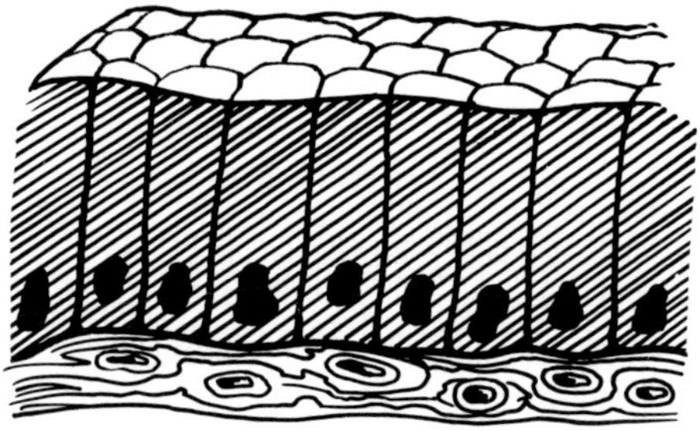

Blood vessels just below the surface.

VAGINA

These cells are exposed to abrasion during intercourse and act as a protective layer. Damaged cells are replaced by new ones from below.

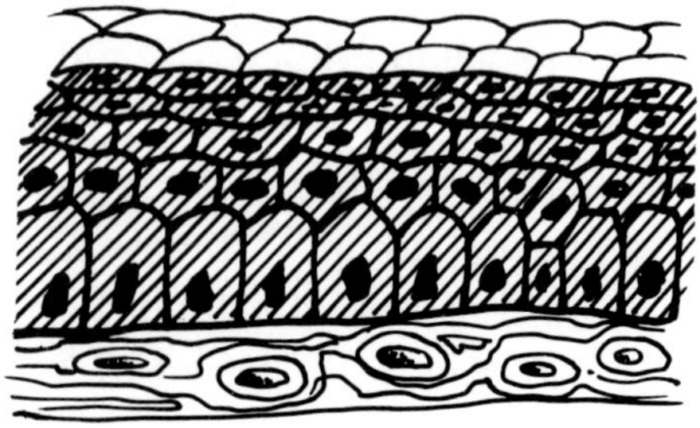

Blood vessels well below the surface.

This two way transmission appears to be happening in Africa and Haiti at the moment but in Europe and America vaginal intercourse does not seem to be a major factor in the spreading of AIDS. In Africa the numbers of infected males and females are almost equal which indicates that heterosexual activity is providing a means of transmission. The reasons are unknown but possibly factors such as malnutrition and the relatively high incidence of other venereal diseases are involved. In Europe and America approximately 95% of all AIDS patients are male.

Moreover, the incidence of AIDS and other sexually transmitted diseases is far higher among homosexual men than any other identifiable group and it would seem that AIDS has spread from America into Europe mainly through homosexual contact.

It is the sexual behaviour of homosexual and bisexual men that makes them the major high risk group, accounting for almost 90% of all AIDS cases. In contrast to other sexually transmitted diseases, it seems that repeated exposure to the AIDS virus is needed to cause infection. The large number of sexual contacts typical of this high risk group can give such exposure: in some cases there can be dozens of sexual partners in a single year.

Predictably there are different levels of risk associated with different sexual activities. Anal intercourse, where the penis enters the rectum,carries the highest possible risk factor. It is risky because in all cases of anal intercourse there is tearing and bleeding of the walls of the rectum. The lining of the rectum is delicate and richly supplied with arteries and veins. Rectal trauma or damage results in the direct mixing of blood and semen. The blood vessels which lie closest to the thin inner lining of the rectum are packed with lymphocytes. If the AIDS virus is present, it will readily invade these cells. While both partners are potentially in contact with the AIDS virus, it is the passive partner, the one receiving the penis, who is most at risk.

Promiscuous anal sex, for many health reasons, is one of the riskiest practices known and carries by far the greatest chance of passing on AIDS if one of the partners has the virus. It is of course entirely possible to contract AIDS from a one night stand with a partner from a high risk group.

Oral or manual stimulation of the anus or rectum should be avoided. Any sexual practice which results in the rupturing or tearing of skin or breaking of blood vessels anywhere on the body is considered to be high risk since it increases considerably the opportunities the virus has for entering the body.

Stimulation of the male or female genitals by the mouth or tongue is also risky, especially if there are cuts or sores or if there is an exchange of semen with an infected partner.

The high risks involved in the exchange of body fluids are predictably compounded by having multiple sexual partners. The same is of course true for all other sexually transmitted diseases.

While kissing is generally thought to be safe, intimate and prolonged kissing with an infected partner must carry some slight risk if there is any bleeding from gums or sores.

No-one has caught AIDS from partners caressing or masturbating, so these may be considered low risk or safe sexual activities.

Intravenous drug users

Apart from homosexual and bisexual males, those most at risk from AIDS are intravenous drug users. These are people who have become so addicted to drugs such as heroin, cocaine and amphetamines that they can satisfy their cravings only by injecting a solution of the drug directly into their veins.

The addicts particularly liable to contract the AIDS virus are those who share their injections with others. They account for about 10% of AIDS cases in Europe at the moment but this figure is rising alarmingly in certain areas.

Some drug users meet in abandoned buildings – the so-called shooting galleries – where illegal drugs are bought and injected intravenously. As many as 50 people might receive injections from the same unsterilised needle. This is a very dangerous activity since it creates the potential for mass infection not only of AIDS but also of hepatitis B, a serious liver disease, and of septicaemia or blood poisoning.

The life-style of many addicts is unhealthy and often they do not take adequate care of themselves. Once they contract AIDS, their immunity to any existing infections they may have is severely reduced.

There is a direct and positive relationship between the number of injections and an addict's chances of catching AIDS. Smoking, sniffing and swallowing drugs are less risky than injecting them, although any illegal drug-taking poses considerable dangers to health. The sharing of any equipment, including the spoons or bowls used for mixing up the drugs prior to injection, is also known to be dangerous. The same is true for tatooing equipment, ear-piercing devices and acupuncture needles, since the exchange of infected blood is possible.

Prostitution involving either males or females is frequently used as a means of paying directly or indirectly for more drugs. (To feed a heroin habit can cost around £40 a day). The sexual partners of such drug users have been known to become infected with the AIDS virus.

Haemophiliacs and people receiving blood transfusions

Haemophiliacs are people who have inherited a genetic disease in which the blood fails to clot because there is a defect in the rather complex clotting process. The disease is characterized by bleeding which may occur spontaneously or after minor tissue damage. The skin, muscles and joints are mainly affected.

The treatment involves immediate pressure to the bleeding sites, followed by transfusions of fresh plasma or of the particular clotting factor which is missing. This treatment may be necessary for a few days. There are several different types of haemophilia depending on which clotting factor is missing; classic haemophilia can be controlled by giving a clotting factor known as Factor VIII. The blood plasma from as many as 20,000 donors may be needed to obtain a single dose. Until recently haemophiliacs who needed large amounts of Factor VIII were particularly at risk from AIDS because some unscreened blood from America had been used in the extraction process. Fortunately the AIDS virus is extremely sensitive to heat and since February 1985 all Factor VIII has been heat treated in order to kill the virus. The risks to haemophiliacs in the UK have therefore been removed, although about 1000 people in the past have received blood or blood products infected with the AIDS virus.

In some countries blood needed for transfusions is not screened for AIDS. Clearly anyone receiving blood from these parts of the world must be considered to be in a high risk group. In the rural clinics of some developing countries, sterilisation of needles and other equipment may also be inadequate.

People who have had sexual contacts in Central Africa

Since AIDS is spreading through the heterosexual community in Central Africa, promiscuous heterosexuals are particularly at risk. In general it appears to be the mobile, affluent town dwellers and female prostitutes who are mainly contracting and transmitting the disease.

Babies born to mothers infected with the virus

Tragically a mother who is carrying the virus can pass it on to her child, either before or after it is born. There are an increasing number of cases where babies have been born already carrying the AIDS virus. In nearly all of them the mother had been infected previously, and the virus passed on across the placenta. Most of the mothers were drug users, and others had been infected by their partners during sexual intercourse. In one or two cases it has been suggested that the virus may possibly have been passed on via the breast milk.

The sexual partners of anyone in a high risk group

Any exchange of body fluids, especially those of blood or semen can result in transmission of the AIDS virus. As with all sexually transmitted diseases, the more partners involved then the greater the risk, be they homosexual or heterosexual. Sexual intercourse with anyone from a known AIDS high risk group will greatly increase that partner's chances of acquiring the disease.

Other risks and fears

Dentists have received advice on the precautions needed to prevent the spread of AIDS from patient to patient or to themselves. It is the bleeding which results from some dental treatment which has caused most concern, rather than the contact with saliva.

Once the immune system is suppressed the tissues of the mouth are highly susceptible to infection by viruses, bacteria and fungi. People with AIDS can have a variety of warts, ulcers and cancers in their mouths. Microscopic bleeding can occur around the gums when the teeth are cleaned and so sharing of toothbrushes is to be avoided. Razors too can become contaminated with infected blood so they are best not shared either.

There has been no evidence so far relating blood-sucking insects such as mosquitoes with the spread of AIDS, probably because the amounts of blood involved are too small.

Furthermore it is most unlikely and so far unknown for anyone to catch AIDS through general social contact, such as shaking hands, touching or embracing someone with AIDS. Nor is it thought that it is in any way possible to catch the disease from lavatory seats, swimming pools, dirty cups, drinking glasses, cutlery or communion chalices. Such myths are typically widespread and have little factual basis. They serve only to further misunderstanding and prejudice.

6. Avoiding AIDS

As the disease has spread through the population and more and more people have become infected, much attention has been directed towards the control and prevention of AIDS. At present there are no anti-viral drugs which are permanently effective against AIDS and no vaccine is in sight. Ways of controlling the infection are therefore strictly limited.

Education is the key, primarily of those in the high risk groups and the related professionals. But education of the general public is also a vital part of the campaign and here the media has a significant role to play in presenting the facts accurately, giving advice on how infection can be avoided and informing people about safer sexual practices.

Over recent decades a freer, more tolerant society has emerged. People have become more open and less sexually inhibited. However there are fears that today's permissiveness has resulted in a trivialisation of human sexual relationships and that this has had a destabilising effect on pair-bonding, marriage and family life. Others see the causes of social ills in a materialistic society which thrives on dissatisfaction and ambition.

Young people today face enormous sexual pressures and expectations. Newspapers, magazines, films, advertisements, radio and television focus ever more heavily and directly on human sexuality. Some feel that this has been partly responsible for an increase in promiscuous behaviour and that the AIDS epidemic is not merely a matter of public health, but intrinsically a moral issue. Some church leaders have suggested that a radical shift in attitudes will be needed to halt the advance of the epidemic.

At the same time there has been wider acceptance in recent years of a simpler, healthier life-style. Deep-rooted habits of over-eating, smoking, and taking little or no exercise are slowly changing.

Nevertheless many feel that to expect society to change its sexual habits – whether for reasons of morality or self-interest – is naive and unrealistic and that a vaccine is the only effective long term answer.

As the virus is transmitted mainly through sexual contact, reducing the number of partners will reduce the chances of contracting the disease. Stable, faithful partners run virtually no risk from AIDS, be they homosexual or heterosexual. Monogamy is by far the safest sexual practice.

However there are many who, for various reasons, reject the concept and practice of monogamous stable pair-bonding, and for a few, especially males, sex has become a sport, largely separate from any deeper emotional involvement.

Those concerned with health care are frustrated by

the reluctance of these groups to appreciate the very real risks they may face. Despite Government efforts, the feeling that "It can't happen to me" is still widespread. If the tide of the epidemic is to be stemmed in the absence of an effective vaccine, then attitudes and expectations must alter, especially among young people.

In a recent survey of public opinion (February 1987), over 80% of those questioned did not consider themselves at risk, and 90% did not expect to have to change their sexual habits.

It is perhaps partly a reflection of the fact that for many years infectious venereal diseases, such as gonorrhoea and syphilis, have been effectively treated and therefore no longer threaten our sexual behaviour.

The condom, also known as the sheath or French letter, has received much publicity in recent months as the most reliable and effective method of protection during either vaginal or anal intercourse. It is one of the simplest and most easily available forms of contraceptive. It consists of a tube of very thin rubber latex, which is rolled over the erect penis just before intercourse. The rubber from which most condoms are made is designed to prevent the penetration of sperms but probably also acts as a barrier to invading microbes. The AIDS virus is 25 times smaller than a human sperm but it is rather fragile and may well be unable to survive passing through the pores of the rubber. The supporting evidence is not extensive and the subject is being more widely researched at present. It is generally accepted however that a condom is less reliable during anal sex, as it is more likely to burst or come off.

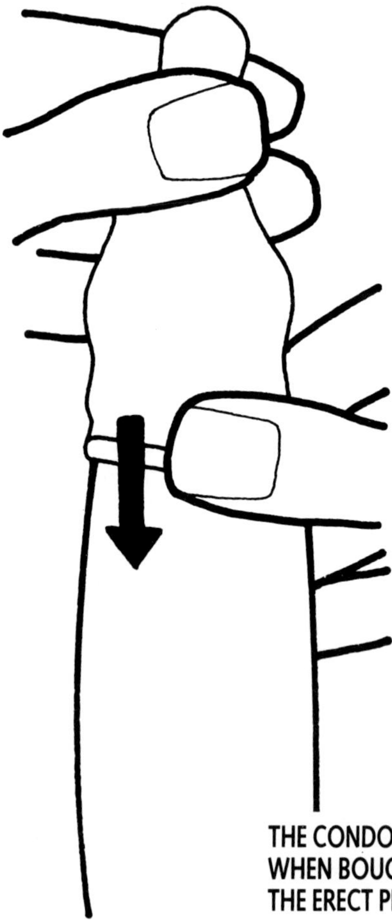

THE CONDOM IS ALREADY ROLLED UP WHEN BOUGHT. IT IS UNROLLED OVER THE ERECT PENIS PRIOR TO INTERCOURSE.

In using a condom it is important that only water-based lubricants are used, since vaseline and other oil-based lubricants may weaken and dissolve the rubber. For full protection, it is also important that the condom is fitted when the penis is hard and erect, before it enters the vagina (or anus) and not just before the moment of ejaculation. This is because some semen leaves the penis before the full orgasm.

Soon after ejaculation, the penis and condom should be extracted together. Once the penis becomes soft or flaccid again, the condom can very easily slide off as it is being withdrawn from the vagina, so care is needed. The condom and its contents should then be disposed of. Spermacides – chemicals to kill sperms – may also be used with condoms and there is some laboratory evidence which suggests they are partially effective against the AIDS virus.

In recent years, other methods of contraception have rendered the condom rather unfashionable but the present advantages of barrier sex should restore its popularity.

Effective counselling and education of those in the high risk groups will play an essential part in controlling the spread of the disease.

Some feel that screening for the presence of the AIDS virus is an important part of controlling the epidemic. At the moment there is no easy test which positively identifies the virus itself. However there is a blood test which fairly easily and reliably identifies the presence of the anti-AIDS virus antibodies.

When a virus or any other microbe enters the body, specific antibodies are produced to fight off the infection. Some antibodies destroy the invading microbe, but unfortunately the HIV antibody does not destroy the virus which causes AIDS. The presence of the antibody shows that at some time that person has been infected with the virus. Such 'antibody positive' people may go on to develop AIDS.

One thing is certain, antibody positives are potentially infective and can pass the virus on to others through unsafe and high risk practices. Whether they themselves will eventually die from AIDS remains uncertain. The figures available vary considerably and it will be some time before a precise picture emerges. So far the majority of antibody positives who take care of themselves have remained fit and well, although the balance seems to be slowly changing against their favour.

Over 95% of patients infected with the AIDS virus have detectable antibodies in their blood. There are at least five different ways of testing for the antibodies. If a blood sample gives a positive result with one test it is then double-checked and confirmed by using another technique. The tests most often used are reliable, require relatively simple equipment, and can be carried out in a couple of working days.

A negative result means that there are no AIDS antibodies in the blood, which probably means that there is no infection. However it can take up to three months for the body to develop antibodies after the virus has invaded. It is therefore important for antibody negatives from high risk groups to be re-tested at regular intervals.

The decision to have the test is a very difficult one and requires great courage. Coping with the result may require more. Here sensitive counselling and strong support are essential.

There are two situations in particular when a test would be very important:

1. It is known that the AIDS virus can pass across the placenta to the unborn child. Any woman at risk, who is or who wishes to become pregnant ought to consider seriously having the antibody test. Such information is necessary for the protection of the baby and of the mother. There is also some fear that if an antibody positive becomes pregnant, she is more likely to develop AIDS. Counselling here must include some discussion on the possibility of abortion.

2. In some cases the antibody test could provide essential and possibly life-saving information in the diagnosis and treatment of an illness.

Ultimately, the decision whether to have a test is highly personal: for some it may be better not to know but for others the uncertainty can be destructive and destabilising. It is very important however that all people in high risk groups, whoever they are, be counselled effectively, regardless of whether they have the antibody test or not.

Until a vaccine is discovered, controlling the spread of AIDS will be achieved only through the adoption of safer sexual practices which take account of the threat posed by AIDS, and by avoiding the abuse of drugs by injection and the sharing of needles and syringes.

Already counselling within the homosexual communities has resulted in a significant decline in the numbers now developing AIDS. Effective counselling of intravenous drug addicts has proved much more difficult. Their perception of life and its values has become so distorted by the drugs to which they are addicted, that sensible advice is often hard to accept, let alone put into action. Some are able to adopt a healthier life-style and give up using drugs altogether. This can be a very hard thing to do, but the encouragement and support of lovers, family and friends can help enormously. For many it is easier to stop fixing whilst continuing to take the drugs in other ways. Those who feel they are unable to change the way in which they take drugs can at the very least avoid sharing equipment, as this involves a special risk of

AIDS infection.

In order to control the spread of AIDS, it is important to protect others in the community. It is therefore essential that all those, even remotely identified as belonging to a high risk group, should ***NEVER*** donate blood, plasma, sperm, or any body tissue or organ. Nor should they ever be shaved at the hairdressers, share razors or toothbrushes. Tattooing, ear-piercing and acupuncture should also be avoided.

The blood and semen of anyone carrying the AIDS virus is potentially infective. These people must accept the very deep responsibility they have for protecting others, whether it be their lovers, with whom they will have intimate contact, or just the friends with whom they share a flat. They all deserve the same degree of honesty.

Once a positive antibody test has been confirmed, not only is there the problem of coping with the possibility of getting AIDS, but also coming to terms with the way other people react. There are many who will be frightened and hostile in their reaction, unwilling to appreciate what it really means to be antibody positive. Others may be more understanding, showing concern and sympathy.

Antibody positives face various problems, including difficulty in getting dental treatment, mortgages, and life insurance. It is important that these people do not become social lepers, rejected by their communities, and it should always be borne in mind that AIDS is not transmitted during the general contact of day to day living.

7. The Care of AIDS Patients

The emotional effect on people confirmed as antibody positive can be devastating and result in profound psychological dependence upon those closest to them. AIDS patients have to come to terms with deep-seated fears of disease, disability, and death. There is also the terrifying prospect that unwittingly they may have passed on the infection to family and loved ones. In addition to this burden they may have to cope with the rejection and prejudice which many in society show towards homosexuals and drug addicts.

As the disease progresses, the need for special physical care and treatment becomes more obvious. Anyone caring for AIDS patients must be reassured that there is no personal risk so long as they are familiar with and follow the appropriate infection control measures. Dealing with spillages of body fluids, such as blood, vomit, urine and semen, requires particular care because these substances can be dangerous when handled carelessly. In all cases rubber gloves should be used to prevent any exposure to the virus, and eye protection and aprons may also be necessary. Whenever possible, the body fluids should be cleared up by the person who produced them and flushed away down the toilet.

If any body fluids from an AIDS patient splash onto someone else's skin, they should be removed immediately with soap and water. Any surface, such as a table or floor, which becomes contaminated should be cleaned with household bleach, freshly diluted 1:10 in water. Where practical the bleach should be left for thirty minutes before being wiped up. Clothes or linen stained with blood, semen or any other body fluid will need to be washed at 95 degrees centigrade. In other areas normal, sensible hygiene precautions are advisable and customary measures such as equipment sterlization should be observed.

Generally AIDS patients do not need to be isolated. However some isolation may be essential for the protection of others if the condition deteriorates considerably and there is incontinence, mental disturbance, bleeding and vomiting.

During the progression of the illness, the needs of the patient will change. In the early stages the patient may be admitted to hospital on several occasions for the treatment of some of the more acute infections. Between these periods he or she may be able to lead a normal life. Later during the course of the disease the precise treatment will depend upon how severe the infections or cancers have become. The physical state of the patient will be a significant factor: with continual chronic diarrhoea and vomiting, malnutrition can often result. The drugs used to treat some of these symptoms can also have unpleasant side-effects.

The basic material needs of AIDS patients are the same, regardless which stage of the disease they have reached. Hygiene is a major priority. Food must be carefully prepared so as to prevent any possible gastro-intestinal infection, to which they are particularly susceptible. Thorough washing of the skin is important to prevent invasion and attack by bacteria and fungi. Mouth infections are common in AIDS patients and therefore good oral hygiene is vital. They should also be protected from exposure to the common cold and 'flu viruses.

A well-balanced diet, rich in protein and vitamins, will help to promote good health and whenever possible some exercise should be taken. Relaxation and rest are also important aspects of patient care.

Most patients suffering from the symptoms of a disease appreciate time and sympathy from their friends and loved ones. When people are terminally ill, their need for affection and friendship is particularly acute. Physical contact, such as holding hands or giving them a hug, can be very reassuring. Friends' willingness to listen to their fears and anxieties may help them to cope with the intense emotional reaction of hopelessness, anger and guilt.

AIDS patients need our compassion, understanding and support to ease their suffering.

8. The Development of a Vaccine

An enormous research effort is currently attempting both to find an AIDS vaccine and to develop or discover a drug which might arrest and defeat the virus once inside the body. Since the discovery of antibiotics in the 1940's, many bacterial infections have been successfully treated with drugs such as penicillin and tetracyclin. These chemicals kill the bacteria and so help the body to fight off the disease. Viruses present much more of a problem as antibiotics are ineffective against them and the body has to depend almost entirely upon its own defences.

So far no drug has been found which will kill any virus, not even one as common as the cold virus. The antiviral drug AZT has had some success in suppressing the reproduction of the AIDS virus, but it seems to be only a short term solution, effective mainly in the early stages of the disease. A major drawback of such antiviral drugs is that severe anaemia may result from their inhibiting effect upon the production of red blood cells.

There are many other difficulties to overcome in fighting the AIDS virus. Not only does it grow and multiply inside the body cells themselves, which makes it hard to get at, but it also infects the brain, so any drug, to be effective, must be able to cross the blood/brain barrier. Another major problem is how to repair and restore the damaged immune system.

Extensive drug trials are under way in America using cultures of ultrasensitive human cells infected with the AIDS virus. The objective is to find a drug which can effectively stop the virus from killing these cells. However there are limitations to such tissue culture techniques. A drug which works well in a test tube may be totally inappropriate for use in the body. It may be toxic or poisonous to many body cells, either immediately or in the longer term. Different cells of the body may react to a drug in a variety of ways. A drug may not be able to reach certain parts of the body, thus allowing the virus to escape unharmed.

In any event the testing of a new drug will have to be exhaustive, so as to eliminate as many uncertainties as possible.

A vaccine is a relatively harmless substance which, when injected into the body, stimulates the production of antibodies. The presence of these specific antibodies means that when the real or harmful form enters the body, there is already an army of antibodies waiting to attack.

Some vaccines, like polio, use a weakened form of the live virus, but this is thought to be far too risky with the AIDS virus.

One approach under investigation uses protein fragments from the outer coat of the AIDS virus. When the protein fragments are injected, they trigger some of the lymphocytes to release specific antibodies which destroy them. These lymphocytes have become 'sensitised' and gradually their numbers increase. If the AIDS virus then enters the body, there is already an army of lymphocytes specially programmed to produce anti-AIDS antibody and the virus will be destroyed.

A major difficulty with the AIDS virus is that it is highly variable. Its genetic structure and outer coating of protein change rapidly, which means that a vaccine giving protection against one form may not provide immunity against others.

Any vaccines must ultimately be tested on humans. Some preliminary results have been obtained using monkeys but this has not been entirely satisfactory since monkeys react differently to the AIDS virus and do not develop the disease. The chimpanzee is the best animal model but there are too few in the world and it is rightly a protected species.

Some feel that in this high-risk, time-pressured situation there is sufficient justification for prescribing the drug directly to humans if trials on monkeys are successful. Others consider such haste irresponsible.

The best answer lies in the production of a live vaccine. With dead vaccine or protein, the body will only respond to the actual amount of chemical put into the body. But living cells will multiply and therefore make the whole process more efficient.

The most recent work involves some skilful genetic engineering. The idea is to take some genetic material from the core of the AIDS virus and transfer it into another virus known to be harmless to humans. The host virus being used in this research is the adenovirus which is large enough to take the extra genes.

The principle is that whilst remaining harmless, AIDS virus protein will form part of the outer coat, and the host virus will multiply inside the body. In response anti-AIDS antibody will be produced: should the AIDS virus attack, the antibodies are ready and waiting. Dogs are being used in current trials to test this technique.

The chances of finding a vaccine are promising, and certainly there is no shortage of ideas. At the moment vaccine trials are being planned in both America and Zaire. One of them, it has been reported, is based upon the vaccine that was used to eradicate smallpox. In Paris a brave group of research workers have injected themselves with trial anti-AIDS vaccine. The stakes in AIDS research are exceptionally high since major discoveries attract considerable scientific kudos and financial reward. However in spite of the urgency it may well take some years before an effective vaccine is widely available.

Already there are an estimated ten million people in the world infected with the AIDS virus, five million in Africa alone. For these people and for those yet to be infected a vaccine is their only hope.